The Patient's Guide

MW01274700

The Patient's Guide

The Patient's Guide in any healthcare setting and during every formal or informal meeting with medical professionals, will help you to:

- Ask useful, concise questions

- Listen, respond and think clearly

- Be brave when at the same time you may be feeling frightened or even helpless

- See the doctor/health professional as an accessible human being

- Establish yourself as an individual

- Be aware of who knows what

- Find your way in often complex health systems

- Make well informed decisions

Jessie Gordon

THE PATIENT'S GUIDE

• • • • • • • • • • • • • • • • •

Think Clearly

Ask Questions

Know People Are
Listening To **You**

PAC-CARD

This book has been written with the aim to help patients and their friends use the PAC-CARD.

The questions on the PAC-CARD (Patient's Action Communication-CARD) are a guide. It is at the end of this book and is available in 8 different languages (date of publication) **as a free download** from **www.pac-card.com**.

The aim of the card and this book is **To Help** the patient feel the right to ask useful questions to any and every Medical Professional in a hospital or other healthcare setting, during all meetings, appointments or interactions.

It is a **Repeatable Checklist** of points to remember. The questions on the card are intended to be asked by the patient, in such a way that the Medical Professionals can either answer them, inform the patient where they may be able to find an answer or simply acknowledge they cannot provide the answer. This book will help you to do this.

It is a simple structure that creates a way of thinking to encourage clear open and time efficient communicaton.

Contents

How to Use This Book

Life is full of surprises. Ranging from the heights of heavenly pleasure to the depths of shock, pain, disbelief. How boring it would be if every day was all on one emotional level and completely predictable! And yet when it comes to our physical health who would not choose a predictably healthy life with no illnesses, no accidents, no surprises?

During the summer of 2007, whilst on holiday in Spain I slipped, fell and broke my ankle, badly. The moment before I fell was insignificant. As far as I was aware, I was taking no physical risks. Just happily walking along a country road, on a sunny summer's day. This accident led to me having surgery with a five-day hospital stay in Spain. Then on my way home through France, I was looked after by several medical professionals and during the next year, back in Amsterdam where I live, I had to make regular visits to hospitals. My whole journey back to health took more than 12 months including a second emergency trip to the hospital in Holland with a blood clot (embolism) in my lung.

Over this whole period I had many meetings with different doctors, nurses and other health specialists. The wide range of these people's communication skills was remarkable. I was grateful to those who listened well, were informed and talked in a way that I could understand. I was all too often distressed, angered and confused by poor communication, both with me and between those around me.

Almost every friend, colleague or acquaintance that I talked with about this, had similar stories of frustration and even despair; the hospital, culture or country made little difference.

One recurring problem seemed to be how helpless, frightened and unintelligent we, the patients, would become, when faced with our own poor health in combination with entering a hospital or medical facility. This personal insecurity would then continue to increase when talking with the Medical Professionals, who of course had a wide range of personalities and communication competencies. The only constant was our self and yet that self, which we knew and generally relied on, was ill or injured.

It became clear to me that to attempt to improve individual doctors' and Medical Professionals' communication skills, as well as hospital communication protocol, was a vast and impossible task. But what I could do in these emotionally charged situations, was attempt to improve my own communication skills. Make myself not only brave but also mentally clear enough to ask the best questions and find out the necessary information to guide my own journey back (hopefully) to health.

Over recent years I have noticed that more and more hospitals provide pamphlets with lists of specific questions for patients to ask, connected to their particular health problem. These are very helpful and I would definitely advise anyone to find out if such a list is available for their particular health problem. But with or without the specific list provided by a hospital or clinic, we the patients need, at any time and in any situation, to be able to navigate the tricky structures and complex relationships of health systems.

Effective communication is vital not only in meetings with the important specialist, but in every interaction we have with any health professional. We the patients are the only ones who will be present at each interaction.

We can never be sure that all the specialists and other practitioners we see will be in full communication with each other. So the more articulate and pro-active we remain the better we will fare. I have experienced that when the patient is clear and as mentally strong as possible then the Health Professionals are also able to do their jobs better. In turn they will feel more fulfilled as they use their training and experience to its optimum. In this way, even during confronting challenging and painful situations, strangely enough there can be pleasure and even satisfaction.

After many conversations with patients and friends, and encouraged by a positive response from Dr R.W. Poolman (my orthopedic surgeon), I collated the PAC-CARD (Patient's Action Communication Card) and set up the website **www.pac-card.com** which offers a free download of the contents of the card. On the website the PAC-CARD is gradually being translated into many languages, at present it is in: Dutch, English, French, German, Portuguese BR, Portuguese PT, Spanish and Turkish. It is offered as a free download card to anyone who wishes to use it. The questions on the PAC-CARD focus on helping the patient to think and talk clearly, listen well, gather information and stay on top of decision-making in situations where they will often feel like the least qualified person in the room. It is a personal support system to develop effective ways of communicating, any time, any place – whatever the pressure.

Dr Poolman was particularly enthusiastic that this guide for effective patient/health professional communication came from a patient. He believed that in this way it would not contain any hospital, doctor or insurance company bias or subtext.

During 2011/2012 a pilot clinical trial assessing the effectiveness of the PAC-CARD was set up by Jeanet Rooseman, Vanessa Scholtes and Dr R.W. Poolman in Onze Liefe Vrouw Gasthuis (OLVG), a large hospital in Amsterdam, the Netherlands. The following was concluded:

'The primary analysis with regard to patient satisfaction in patient-caregiver communication showed that the PAC-CARD had a positive impact on two aspects of patient satisfaction in the intervention group. Patient satisfaction regarding quality of care and the way of communication improved significantly in the intervention group.

To support patients in a more structured way of communicating the PAC-CARD is recommended to be used by patients. It helps patients communicate more effectively and patients are more satisfied with the quality of care and communication.'

This book will give you tips on how best to use the PAC-CARD which is printed at the end of this publication. It will also include a background to the ideas, real life examples (sometimes a person's name for the sake of privacy has been changed) and additional tips plus some empty pages for you to note down thoughts, questions and information as you read the book. The PAC-CARD will act as a checklist to remind and support you at moments when it is so easy to forget. It will help you to counterbalance high emotion such as fear with intelligent curiosity. So you can become your own **private investigator**, getting the best out of all the health professionals. Assume that they want to help you, even if it does not always feel that way.

The questions on the card are intended to be asked, by you the patient, in such a way that the health professional does not feel criticized or attacked but is stimulated to either answer the question or simply acknowledge they cannot provide an answer. This book will also give you some tips on how to do this.

Some fairly straightforward questions seem to become impossible, over-demanding or even rude when put in a medical context . But after a while you will get used to asking the PAC-CARD questions. The PAC-CARD will help you become familiar with asking normal questions in an unfamiliar environment where one can so easily feel powerless and stupid.

You do not have to use all of the points on the PAC-CARD during every interaction. They are there to remind and help you to:

- **Establish yourself as an individual, not an illness.**
- **See the doctor/health professional as a human being.**
- **Be brave when at the same time you may be feeling frightened, in pain and even helpless.**
- **Listen well and think clearly.**
- **Ask useful, concise questions.**
- **Keep on finding out who knows what.**
- **Navigate a health system which – as in any organization run by people – will make mistakes.**

No one can look into the future. Each decision or action we take is a calculated guess. Sometimes the guesswork can evolve into a feeling that we can indeed predict the future. We even demand and expect this from the experts. These expectations of certainty can easily lead to frustration, disappointment and anger. From the point of view of the doctor these negative feelings can happen as they feel pushed into promising something that deep down they know they can never be 100% sure of. And from the point of view of us, the patients, if it does not go the way we hoped for or the doctor promised we can become increasingly insecure and frightened.

All any of us can do is remain as informed and alert as possible in order to be able to make the next best decisions – intelligent guessing.

Feel free to read and re-read this book in any way you wish. It is here to support and remind you of ways to think and communicate effectively within a medical environment. You can turn to any section which is relevant to your immediate needs or just start at the beginning and work your way through all the ideas in the book. Make it your own personal 'travel guide'.

In this book instead of individually referring to doctors, surgeons, nurses, specialists, therapists – i.e. any person who has an expertise and training in the medical profession – I will often use the collective term: Health Professional.

Each chapter number links to the same number on the PAC-CARD checklist.

1. Take Someone With You

To listen and really hear what someone is telling us about our own health, let alone be able to discuss this information, is for most of us surprisingly hard to do.

This may be because of either physical pain and exhaustion, emotional pain or both. Some of the emotions which are pretty common on such occasions are anticipation, confusion, fear, anger, panic. These emotions will easily stimulate a physical reaction in the body in the form of adrenaline. Adrenaline is one of the chemicals which creates the fight or flight response. It makes the heart beat faster, preparing the body to react to danger. The side effects can, for example, make you feel too hot or too cold, have sweaty and shaking hands, a dry mouth, a tight feeling in the throat or even have a desire to vomit. With some people an adrenaline rush can sharpen their mind, with others it can cloud it. But whatever your particular reaction to an adrenaline rush is, it is unlikely that you will be able to think in the same way as you would for example if you were relaxing at home with friends.

1a. Whenever possible, it is useful to have someone with you who knows you and can also remain objective.

In any situation where we are trying to understand, remember and respond to important information it helps to have the support of someone who knows and understands us. If we are under pressure it becomes even more important. In such meetings it is all too easy to forget to ask even the most obvious or pressing question.

This is why we need an ally to help us think clearly, listen well and ask all the questions we wish and need to ask. This is practical and for some people may be easy to arrange. But if we have many medical appointments or maybe are admitted to hospital, then it may not feel like such a simple thing to do.

For outpatient appointments some people may have a partner or friend who is always available and willing to come along. Although we may feel uncomfortable with regularly asking someone to come with us, we should not underestimate the benefits – and not only to ourselves.

For us the patients, it will not only help us to listen to the information and discuss it. It will also mean that if we feel pain or have emotions which, during the conversation, prevent us from hearing or thinking clearly, we will know that later we will be able to discuss the content of the meeting with our friend or partner.

The Health Professional will be able to continue to discuss the possible courses of treatment or symptoms without us having to contain our feelings or think logically. In this way we can proceed without the meeting having to be stopped or rescheduled.

For our friend(s) and/or partner it means that they will be more empowered to help us, think along and add their perspective in our life together. After the meeting we will be able to discuss what took place with someone we know well who was actually there, and as we all hear and understand differently, with their added perceptions we will be more informed. Most people will be confronted with health problems at some point in their life. By including others and daring to ask for help it is an act of trust in your relationship as well as giving them time to remember their own relationship with health.

It will also mean that we are less likely to become isolated with our health problem.

Sometimes it will just not be practical or possible to have a friend or partner with us. In this case we can try to enlist someone else as our ally.

For example, if you are in a hospital ward and there are other people sharing the room with you, see if you can get to know them a little. There may be someone who has a similar illness to yours or at least who you can have some kind of empathy with. When the medical staff come round each day to discuss your progress you could ask the fellow patient to listen in and think along with you.

Alternatively it may be that you 'click' with one of the nursing staff, and that you specifically ask them if, once the doctor has seen you, you can double check your understanding of the latest information with them.

Tony R. was in hospital recovering from a small operation. In his ward was a young woman in her early 30s, Ingrid T., who had just had her tonsils removed. She was due to be discharged from hospital that afternoon and was worrying that with the amount of pain she was experiencing, she would not be able to cope with her two young children, once she got home. She wanted to stay another 24 hours in the hospital to recover a bit more.

Because she was in so much pain, without thinking too clearly about who would be the best person to discuss her concerns, she asked the nurse on duty if she could stay another day. The nurse (whose decision it turned out it was not hers to make) flatly refused and the two of them ended up in a heated argument.

Tony, because he empathized with Ingrid, having a few years earlier also experienced similar pain with the same operation, tried to intervene. Eventually he found one of the doctors and explained Ingrid's fears and the unfortunate conflict with the nurse. In this case it would have been better to first discuss the request with the doctor. As a patient it is not so easy to understand the decision making structure of your ward or hospital, and if you are in a lot of pain then to find out who to ask what becomes even harder.

A solution was discussed and a compromise was reached. If Ingrid had made an ally of Tony earlier in the day, she might have talked through her fears with him and then had him listen in as she asked the nurse. Even better, she might have realized through discussion that it might be better to first ask who made the decisions concerning a patient being released from hospital. The whole interaction might then have been less upsetting and more efficient.

TIPS – *'Take someone with you'*

* Remember that being brave does not mean trying to cope by yourself.
* It is perfectly normal to need and ask for help from your friends and family.
* Help your friends and family help you, by being clear about when you have appointments – ask for help in good time for them to make arrangements and be available for you.
* Remember that to ask someone for help is a compliment and can be seen as a vote of confidence in your friendship as well as an appreciation of their ability to help you.
* Some people have their own fears around hospitals or similar medical institutions – check to see if this is the case, people can be quite shy about admitting it.
* Try and have a group of people who you can choose from to accompany you to different appointments, so one person does not get overly pressurized either by time commitments or emotional involvement.
* If you have a selection of friends who agree to support you during hospital visits and important medical meetings, let the friends know who is involved so that they can also support each other.

* Be on the look-out for possible allies in the situations where your immediate family or friends cannot be present.
* Be aware and ready to be someone else's ally.

Note: If you are admitted to hospital, whenever possible clearly tell the administration who from your support network of friends and family may have access to your latest medical information. Make sure that your friends and family know who are the main contact people.

1b. Introduce your companion and say that they will be helping you understand, remember the meeting and also ask questions if they need to.

If you introduce your companion it will give a clear indication to the Health Professional that you wish them to take an active part in the conversation. This will also give your companion the authority to be part of the conversation. You may also decide to ask your companion to take notes during the meeting for you. If you discuss the meeting with them beforehand and make a list of topics and questions which you wish to cover, then they can help make sure this happens.

TIPS – *'Introduce your companion...'*

* Introduce your friend/partner as soon as possible at the beginning of any meeting, and add that they are your extra pair of ears and eyes, and when necessary will also be asking questions.

* Remember to ask your companion to include you with any conversation they have with the Health Professional, on your behalf. They can do this by regularly including you with their eyes as they talk.

* Ask your companion to use your name rather than referring to you as 'he ' or 'she' if they are talking about you with the Health Professional.

* You and your companion need to feel like a team. Regular eye contact between you can help this.

* Feel free in the meeting to ask your companion if they have any questions or if you do not understand, check if they do!

* This is not a business meeting. If you feel like the added support of holding hands or even having an arm around you, feel free to ask for it.

2. Give Information To Any Doctor/ Health Professional You Have Not Met Before

Each time we meet someone, we will be drawn into making assumptions about what kind of person they are. This happens very fast and will result in some kind of conclusion: *'Oh he or she is that sort of person.'* These opinions will be arrived at in quite basic ways. They will be connected to assumptions about age, gender, nationality, race, clothes, accent and word use. Physical and vocal communication habits as well as personal preferences and prejudices will also play a part.

People have a tendency to put other people in stereotype boxes. In some instances it can be very useful but sometimes it stops us from seeing and really understanding the other person.

As most meetings with Health Professionals in hospitals are short it is all the more important that within a few sentences you can make sure that the Heath Professional sees YOU, not their assumptions about you, and hears the information you want them to hear.

You are an individual not a sickness.

To make sure that the Health Professional sees and hears YOU, you have to see and hear yourself. This means that though you may be feeling concerned or even overwhelmed by not only your ill-health but also the hospital or clinic, it is important to keep touching base with yourself and your core qualities. Those qualities which in your day-to-day life function perfectly well. This can be done in quite a simple way by pro-actively becoming more aware of a few things:

TIPS – *for 'coming home –into yourself'*
* **Feel the weight of your body under your feet, if you are standing, or under your bottom, upper thighs and feet if you are sitting.**
* **Notice your breath and maybe slow it down (taking 3 longer, deeper, slower breaths inhaling and exhaling).**
* **Be aware of the temperature of the air on your skin.**
* **Notice 2 or 3 different sounds.**
* **Notice where the light is coming from.**
* **Let your jaw and shoulders feel heavy and loose.**

In this way you can come home into your body even when it is not at that moment a great place to be.

You can try this or a similar sequence many times to help move your thoughts away from any possible anxieties.

Then as you meet the new Health Professional, by giving a brief description of yourself you will help them to see you as an individual.

Do not assume they already know:

2a. Your age

It is interesting how often Health Professionals do not register this even if it is noted in your file. They may just make a quick calculation from the way you appear.

My mother in the last year of her life at the age of 89 had several stays in hospital. Since she looked more like she was in her early 70s, each time she declared her age the staff would be amazed, confused and even embarrassed. Of course in some situations to be seen as older or younger than your calendar years can be to your advantage but in a medical context it is important for Health Professional to be accurately informed.

2b. Your profession and education

In a couple of sentences describe your expertise/profession and knowledge base, even if you are not paid money for it, for example as in full time parenting. The Health Professional will then know what kind of references to use as they talk with you. They may talk with a different image for example about a heart problem if they are talking with an electrician, cook, teacher or full time parent.

2c. Your social background

We all have slightly different value systems, and it is useful for the Health Professional to take this into consideration and not just assume for example if I am Chinese that I use acupuncture and am not a Christian. Different cultures and beliefs can have very different approaches to what is or is not acceptable with medical care. It is all too easy to misunderstand and assume. These presumptions can also have an effect on how the Health Professional may diagnose your symptoms.

Zena R. (born in England and living in Holland) was meeting with a new doctor who needed to know which standard blood tests she had recently had. Zena's mother had been born in India, so Zena filled this in on the form her doctor had given her requesting certain background information. But her mother was not Indian. Because Zena had slightly

olive coloured skin, brown eyes and dark hair the
doctor assumed she was half Indian, and enquired
if she had ever been tested for hepatitis B. Zena
was a bit surprised and said no. The doctor then
proceeded to describe the importance of knowing if
she had this virus and the probable likelihood due
to her mother being born and growing up in India.
This misunderstanding went on for about 5 minutes
before Zena realized that the doctor had made
an incorrect assumption about her mother and
her. If Zena had not realized this and challenged
the doctor's conclusion, it could have resulted in
unnecessary anxieties and blood tests.

2d. Tell your recent/relevant medical history including allergies and any medications.

Before most appointments Health Professionals will
not have had enough time to study your complete
medical file, especially if it is long. And even if they
have had a reasonably good look it may not include
the most relevant up-to-date information. You may be
taking a medicine which is not noted in the file they
have access to. With any first meetings it is essential
to quickly give the Health Professional an overview of
important facts concerning recent medical interven-
tions as well as the drugs you may have been on or

are presently taking. It is important to note everything even if you think it is unrelated. For example if you are seeing a specialist for stomach problems and you are also taking eye drops for a minor eye problem let them know. Give Health Professionals the opportunity to decide if the different drugs could affect one another or not. With any allergies you cannot re-state them enough. For example I am allergic to penicillin. Over the years I have noted that this fact will rarely be carried from one file or document to the next.

TIPS – *'Tell your recent/relevant medical history including allergies and any medications.'*

❋ **Make a synopsis of your recent medical history and have it at hand to read out so you do not have to worry about missing out any important facts.**

❋ **As you tell the Health Professional watch their reaction – did they already know what you were telling them? If not, do you see them adding it to your file? If they indicate that they are already informed (be pleased!) quickly move to the next point on your list.**

3. Ask Questions Of Any Doctor/ Health Professional You Have Not Met Before (And Google Them)

Since Health Professionals will have some kind of training and experience in their area of medicine, we the patients will quite reasonably have expectations that they can help us. The more high-ranking they are the more we will tend to expect from them. We will most probably hope that they can solve our medical problems. If they cannot make us better who can?

The amount of pressure put on doctors, surgeons and specialists can be considerable. During their career there will be many times when they do perform amazing acts of diagnosis and surgery, often prolonging or saving a patient's life as well as improving a patient's health-related quality of life. There will also be times when, despite their years of training and experience, they can do little or nothing to cure the patient or alleviate their pain.

Maybe because little emphasis is put on communication skills during many doctors' trainings, their abilities to interact with their patients vary widely. There also seems to be little training related to helping doctors to deal with fear and anxiety – both their own and their patients'.

So what can happen is that the patient turns the doctor into some kind of demi-god who can and should make them better, and the doctor to emotionally protect themselves adopts an aloof, god-like attitude towards the patient. However, I have noticed that over the past 10 years this is beginning to shift (slightly!).

By asking the doctor a few simple questions about themselves we can help to remind everyone in the room that we are all human. They are a human being with a lot of expertise, but nevertheless human and imperfect!

3a. How long have they worked here and what is your role/function?

As much as it is useful for a Health Professionl with a few short questions to get an idea about us the patient, it can also help us understand what they say if we know a bit about them. *For example: if I am meeting with an orthopedic surgeon to discuss an operation to correct a bunion on my big toe, if I know that he specializes in backbone re-constructions then clearly from his point of view, my foot surgery is a minor operation. He may even joke about it!* So questions like: *"What is your specialty?", "How long have you worked at this hospital?"* and *"What is your function within this hospital?"* can not only help us to know what to expect from them, but can also allow the doctor to show themselves to the patient as a human with certain interests and a particular expertise, rather than just a title.

Sometimes we may not even be in the same room as the Health Professional. If we do not know who they are it is important to quickly know what their title/experience is so that we can decide what to do with the information they give us. As in the case of Gerda.

Gerda K. (mid thirties) awoke suddenly at five in the morning with an unbearable headache. It felt as if she was being repeatedly stabbed in her head. She staggered to the toilet, vomited and then had diarrhea. Since her sister had died some years earlier of a stroke from a haemorrhage (bleeding) in the brain, Gerda was already alerted to the fact that there might be this genetic weakness in her family. She therefore immediately rang up the emergency services. Because the pain was severe she could hardly talk or think clearly. Gerda told the person who answered her call that she thought she was either having a heart attack or a stroke. The emergency services receptionist told Gerda she was over-reacting and hyperventilating. She instructed Gerda to breathe slowly using a plastic bag, to calm herself down. She then told Gerda to call her own doctor once the daily surgery opened later that morning. Since Gerda was in so much pain she did not ask the receptionist the simple question: "Could you please tell me what your qualifications are? I would like to know who is giving this advice." In this case it turned out that the person was not a doctor. If Gerda had found out from whom the advice was coming she could then decide if she wanted a second opinion. Several hours later Gerda did get to hospital (she was indeed having a stroke) and was operated on later that day. She survived without any long-lasting damage, in spite of the ill-advised instructions of the emergency services telephonist. Of course we cannot re-write history, but Gerda might have been able to immediately get the ambulance which she urgently needed, if she had asked to talk with someone who could accurately assess her condition.

TIPS – 'How long have you worked here and what is your role/function?'

* Before a first meeting with a doctor, specialist or surgeon, visit the hospital website or do a web search on their name to see what you can find out about them. This will mean that they are already slightly familiar to you. It will also help you to ask relevant questions when you meet them, which will show that you are interested in them and their expertise.

* When asking any of the personal questions of a Health Professional remember to stay curious and non-judgmental – keep in the back of your mind that you want to get to know them a little better, rather than test them out, or interview them for a job!
* If you have not been able to research the Health Professional before meeting with them, these questions are even more valuable.
* Just because a Health Professional may be young or new to the hospital does not mean that they are any less capable.

Hester L. was diagnosed with scleroderma, a rare chronic autoimmune disease. Her way of coping with this was to remain as positive as she could, find the specialist who could best help her and get on with her life. As the condition progressed she needed to regularly see her specialist as well as have telephone appointments to check in with him. The morning before one of the telephone appointments with her specialist Hester's husband noticed that she was particularly unwell. He persuaded her, instead of waiting for the telephone appointment, to go directly to the hospital, his reasoning being: "If the specialist has time to talk with you on the phone for ten minutes he also has ten minutes to see you." When Hester got to the hospital the receptionist was

*unable to arrange for her to see the specialist, but
the specialist offered the possibility to directly meet
with one of the junior doctors. Hester readily agreed.
The junior doctor immediately saw that Hester
needed emergency medical attention. She insisted
that Hester lay down and then alerted the specialist.
Without delay Hester was admitted to hospital. The
fast action of this junior doctor saved Hester's life. A
few weeks later Hester passed the junior doctor in
the corridor of the hospital and was able to thank
her personally. These few words of thanks were a
surprise to the junior doctor and much appreciated!*

3b. Do you have access to all my medical records?

Increasingly a patient's medical file will be in a digital
format. As well as being a more convenient way to
share information, for some it has become a bit of a
tyranny – more and more I hear that during appointments the Health Professional's attention is drawn
towards keeping the file up to date rather than talking
with the patient. Hospitals, clinics and local doctors
increasingly have access to your files. But this is not
always the case. Often a patient's files will be a mix of
different systems, both handwritten and digital, and
often a centralizing file system is not fully functional.
So, although the question may feel insulting, it is ac-

tually a realistic and practical one which could benefit both you and the Health Professional

*J*an W. had broken his leg several weeks earlier and although each day, a couple of hours after waking up, he would have a very swollen leg, foot and ankle it seemed from his regular check-ups that the bones were healing well. They had even put a lighter support plaster on his leg so that his skin had access to the air. One morning he awoke with a stabbing pain in his chest. After about an hour he tried to call his doctor but was put through to a central agency who after hearing his symptoms immediately sent for an ambulance. It turned out that he had an embolism (blood clot) which had lodged itself in his lungs and was life-threatening. He was admitted to the lung department of the hospital, immediately put on blood thinners and luckily survived. Three days later he was discharged from hospital.

Later that same day as he was examining the precise area of the break on his leg he saw that the skin was more swollen than usual and rather warm to the touch. He called his GP (general practitioner), who when she saw Jan's leg immediately arranged for him to return to the hospital to see his orthopedic specialist. That same afternoon as Jan talked with the orthopedic specialist he mentioned his added *concern due to the lung embolism. This was the same hospital, but a different department, and his orthopedic specialist knew nothing about Jan's stay in hospital earlier in the week. With this added information he immediately changed his advice and was much more attentive. Jan was extremely upset and felt very insecure, because he presumed although it was an enormous hospital that the IT system would cross-reference each patient's identity number to all departments and important medical information would be shared. This was not the case. If Jan had just asked the question at the beginning of the appointment rather than assuming that this modern hospital had a cross-referencing system in place, it might have been less upsetting, the doctor could have immediately prescribed the best treatment and time would have been saved.*

If as a matter of course we keep checking with Health Professionals to see what information they have access to we will then know when to fill in the gaps. Or indicate that there is added information which they should or could have access to. With even quite simple complaints or illnesses it can get surprisingly complex as we are sent from one department or clinic to the next for various specialist tests.

✳ **Similarly to the way you ask Health Professionals about themselves, make sure that the way you ask about their access to your files is 'light' and curious. If Health Professionals feel you are policing them they can become defensive and in some extreme cases even unhelpful.**

✳ **Do not let any feelings of insecurity get in the way of regularly asking this question, it could make a big difference to a Health Professional's analysis, recommended treatment and your recovery.**

3c. If I want to see them, how do I get access to my medical records?

I am amazed how many people feel that they do not have the right to look at their own medical file. Whether we understand anything which is written in the file, is quite a different issue! But it is surprisingly empowering to know, should I wish to read the file(s) or show them to someone else, that I know how to get access to this information. Our medical file is ours, and we have the right to read or have a copy of it.

Knowing how to obtain access to our medical file can also be useful. Different institutions and countries have different filing systems, and we may find ourself in a situation when a doctor needs quick access to our main file and does not immediately know which channels to use to make this happen. Not only that but files sometimes get lost. This rarely happens (I hope) but just in my circle of friends I have known of two instances. If we are aware of how a particular institution collates and stores a patient's files, we will have more insight into what information the Health Professional could have, and if it is mislaid...well we could offer them our copy!

Thomas G., 19 years old, was in a car accident and sustained multiple injuries. This resulted in among others a major operation to his lower spine, which had been shattered during the collision. After many months of re-habilitation and several more operations he was able to leave the hospital. At the time he asked if he could take copies of his X-rays with him. This was denied. Twelve years later, due to ongoing back problems, he had a new set of X-rays made (different city, different hospital). The specialist at the second hospital wanted to see the first set of X-rays which had been taken immediately after the accident, and then again after the surgery, in order to compare this information with the present X-rays. The specialist believed it was important to see if anything had changed over the past 12 years and this was the only way she could really analyse this. When Thomas contacted the first hospital they announced that this was not possible as after 10 years their policy was to destroy files which were 'inactive'.

These days most probably a lot of hospital files including X-ray and MRI data will be digital. But this is not necessarily the case. If Thomas had insisted on having his own copy of the X-rays, he could have been sure that they would not be lost.

TIPS – *'If I want to see them, how do I get access to my medical records?'*

* **Decide if you only want to know how to get access to your medical records, should you in the future want to see them, or if you actually want to see the file right now.**
* **There will be degrees of complexity to realizing this request, depending whether the files are multiple, interdepartmental, digital, handwritten...**
* **If permission is denied or the question evaded, ask why.**
* **You do not have to give a reason why you would like to have access to your files. You do not have to defend your position.**

4. Describe Only Your Symptoms

These days with the ease of internet search engines such as Google many of us can instantly have access to extraordinary amounts of information about almost anything. A common reaction when people find out something is wrong with their health is to immediately 'google' the symptoms and see what the online specialists describe and advise. If we are already feeling worried and have little or no medical training then to try to analyse our own symptoms can lead to alarming conclusions! It is easy enough to imagine that we have any number of horrible and strange conditions – very often several symptoms that we may be experiencing will correspond with countless illnesses.

This is not to dismiss the internet completely, it can be extremely useful, but it will be as intelligent as the way we use it.

Maybe because we want to feel less helpless and as informed as each Health Professional we meet, it is common for patients to arrive at an appointment with several possible diagnoses already cooking inside their head! So when the doctor asks us to describe our symptoms we already tell the doctor what we think the symptoms could mean.

The problem with this can be twofold. By trying to fit our symptoms into an illness we have read about we are less likely to notice ALL the actual symptoms we may be experiencing. The different, often subtle signs which our body is giving us are then more likely to be missed by everyone. It is vital that we clearly describe to the specialist the full pattern and array of what is happening to us. In this way they will be more able to truly assess the situation and put their skill and knowledge to work.

Harry B. noticed that he had blood in his stools. First of all he ignored it. Then after several weeks, as it persisted, he went on the internet to try some self-diagnosis. Two illnesses immediately sprang out at him. Firstly colon cancer, and secondly Crohn's Disease – a colleague at work had that and in the end after almost dying, had most of his large intestine removed and now had a colostomy. He could not sleep with the anxiety and fear of what was happening to his body. And when he finally arrived in the doctor's surgery he immediately declared that he either had colon cancer or Crohn's Disease. The doctor tried to get him to calm down, and then asked Harry some questions, including the following: "Have your stools changed colour, if so when did this happen and what was the colour change? How often do you have a bowel movement? What is the consistency? What colour is the blood? Is it bright red and fresh looking or dark brownish to black...?"

Harry could not answer these or any other questions. As the appointment continued it was clear that they could not proceed. Harry needed to come back in a few days with an accurate list of his symptoms before the doctor could even begin to consider what was wrong with him. He spent another few days trying to get a more accurate awareness of his symptoms, all the while feeling frightened and nervous.

It turned out that he was suffering from haemorrhoids, a relatively minor and easily treatable condition.

Secondly, if we the patients immediately suggest a certain diagnosis it can have a variety of negative effects on the Health Professional. They may subconsciously favour our diagnosis, becoming less than objective in their examination of the symptoms, or they may react against *"yet another patient telling me how to do my job"* and discount it as a possible conclusion.

It is worth noting that in some cultures Health Professionals are advised to ask a patient what they think they are suffering from as a structural part of the consultation. If you are asked, and if you have formed an opinion, then naturally you should give it.

Let the Health Professional use their own resources to analyse your individual and unique case. Let them gather all possible information about you and what is happening to you. Listen to what they have to say and use the PAC-CARD questions to guide your conversation. Then if they have not mentioned one of the illnesses or awful conditions you have read about which seem to match most of your symptoms, *'to put your mind at rest'* maybe ask the specialist why according to them you do not have that particular illness!

4a. Make notes before hand to refer to.

TIPS – *'Make notes before hand to refer to'*
* **Make a list beforehand of any symptoms you may be experiencing. Refer to it during your meeting with the Health Professional.**
* **Create this list over a few days or even weeks so you can have a better overview of when certain things happen.**

* Note, what type of activity you are doing, how long the symptoms last plus the frequency, and time of day.
* Note precisely where on your body.
* If pain is involved see if you can give it some kind of grade, and note it down. For example 0–10 (0 = no pain, 10 = unbearable pain)
* If you already have a possible *'condition'* in your mind before you meet the specialist wait until later in the meeting to mention it. Let them know that it is concerning you but also be clear that this diagnosis comes from an amateur's search on, for example the internet.
* If the specialist comes to a similar conclusion to the one you had reached, let them know.
* If you want to know more background information, ask if the specialist can recommend any reliable sources for you to further inform yourself.

5. Discuss All Of The Following During The Meeting

All the questions in this section are there to help guide you through an informative and thoughtful discussion concerning you and your health, with Health Professionals.

It is useful to keep coming back to all the questions in one way or another, depending on who we are talking with. If we regularly use these questions, they will become a familiar and easy tool to support our thinking when we are talking with Health Professionals. The more we can get used to covering and using the full range, the more it will become instinctively apparent to us which question(s) we most need in any given interaction.

5a. What is the problem?

This is the biggest and most urgent question which will be concerning most of us. What is wrong with me? Is it minor or life threatening? Doctor, can I be cured? Will I soon be able to return to my life as if nothing has happened?

Firstly, we need to decide if we really want to know. Sometimes people prefer not to be informed at all and want the doctors to take charge, and hopefully *'make them better'*. This is for each of us to decide. If that happens to be how you would like to proceed by either delegating full responsibility to your doctor, a family member or both it is useful to know this about yourself and to state it early on, in any meeting with Health Professionals. In which case be clear who of your friends or family is the point of reference for the Health Professionals. This is important from both your family's point of view as well as that of the hospital. If you decide to take this path, remember that at any point you can also change your mind and ask to be informed. Sometimes a family member may have to take charge of the situation, as in the case of Caroline.

As Caroline W. was driving her father to the hospital, to get the results of various medical tests, her father was clearly unwell and panicky. Suddenly he announced that if there was anything seriously wrong with him he would rather not know. In fact he did not want to go to the hospital and asked her to immediately turn the car around and drive him back home. Ever since her mother's death the year before Caroline had noticed that her father, who previously had been a strong, independent character, had been visibly crumbling, both emotionally and mentally. He was not dealing at all well with the death of his wife (of 46 years). Caroline very much doubted whether without the support of her mother, if indeed he did have a serious condition, he would be able to cope. However, she managed to persuade her father to come with her to the hospital, since she was herself anxious to know the results of the tests. Before the appointment got under way, Caroline took the attending physician aside and explained her father's state of mind. The physician immediately suggested that Caroline's father went back and waited in the reception area, and then proceeded to discuss her father's symptoms and a possible course of action in his office with Caroline. Because Caroline had been clear before the appointment even started both she and the physician could elegantly navigate this potentially upsetting situation. It turned out that her father was suffering from Parkinson's Disease. Together with the rest of the family and some close friends she was able to support her father through the last years of his life. He never changed his attitude, and remained ignorant of his condition, right up to the day he died. Whenever Caroline or one of her brothers accompanied their father to any kind of medical appointment, they made sure that they all regularly re-stated their father's wish to remain uninformed. It was surprisingly tricky sometimes to maintain this stance as over the years quite a *few Medical Professionals attended him. But by being persistently clear with each and every Medical Professional the family managed to support him in a consistent and elegant way. Later Caroline realized that her father had probably put two and two together and most probably knew what was wrong with him. She thought that maybe his choice was partly due to his desire – conscious or otherwise – to avoid the numerous conversations and decisions which had to be made concerning him and his health.*

By asking *'what is the problem?'* we are not necessarily looking for a definitive diagnosis. We are asking for what is known at that moment in time. It is useful to note how the Health Professional answers this. For example: do they immediately come to a conclusion... give us a list of likely causes... or keep any diagnosis open and vague? The range of answers will be huge depending on what we are suffering from. There is a great difference between discussing a broken arm and cancer. However, even with the most seemingly simple physical complaint there may be different opinions concerning *'what the problem is'*. If you are suffering from a collection of symptoms and this is your first appointment with a specialist, by being clear with this first question you may quickly realize whether this is the specialist you should be consulting or even the hospital you should be visiting.

It is also useful to remember that our health is a changing and complex matter and although in many hospitals we will often visit a specialist for one part of our body or one particular illness, our body is in fact a *team effort*. This means that if you have a wide range of symptoms you may end up visiting a collection of different specialists.

It is not uncommon for specialists to find out what is wrong with someone and how to treat it through a process of trial and error. They may be extremely knowledgeable and experienced, but each patient is a different and unique case. Luckily we will have many similarities with other patients, which is how Health Professionals will be able to make a diagnosis, but the fact still remains that we are all different.

Each Health Professional will tend to look at your health problem from their specific specialist point of view. Because it is highly likely that a patient will have to interact with many Health Professionals *'What is the problem?'* is a very useful question to keep asking, any time, any place...

> When Chris J. broke his ankle he was rushed to hospital. Although he did not know it at the time, it was a very bad break right the way through the two main bones in his leg. The only way he could

bear the pain was by holding his leg out and down
so his foot hung freely. When he was wheeled into
the X-ray department on the wheelchair the nurse,
to be able to do her job well, proceeded to try to get
him to lie on a bed with his leg flat out in front of
him. This was unbearably painful for him. It was not
until he described to her what his problem was with
this position and she explained what her problem
was, that they could come up with a solution. Using a
combination of cushions and the nursing staff helping
Chris to hold a certain strange position completely
still for a few seconds, they were able to make a clear
X-ray, so the doctor could then make a diagnosis.

TIPS – 'What is the problem?'

* With each interaction with Health Professionals
  ask yourself what is the point of the meeting?
  In this way the question *'What is the problem?'*
  will have a clear goal.

* The overriding reason for asking this question
  will be to help you assess how you should proceed
  with any possible actions.

* Keep remembering that any answer to this question
  is part of a process – it is a point of departure.

* When analysing and identifying a certain health
  problem this question will need to be asked many
  times – try not to lose heart.

5b. What can be done?

Whatever a diagnosis may be, whether it is clear-cut or on the path towards finding out more, there will be a point in the discussion when it is useful to identify what action can be taken. It is not until we can list and understand the full range of possible actions that we can even begin to make decisions between one course of action and another. Similar to the question *'What is the problem?'* there will be a large range to the type of action points. It is important to keep asking this question in such a way that we find out not only what that particular specialist and hospital is able to do but what are the full range of possible actions connected to our physical problem (maybe worldwide). Sometimes what is proposed is directly related to financial considerations or what is available depending on time pressure or medical resources. Different doctors will prefer different courses of action. And then if we are going to be cynical we should not underestimate the part drug companies play in encouraging the medical establishment to use their products. I believe that for us the patients it is very hard to find out about that particular subtext, but by simply asking a specialist the broad question of *'What can be done?'* we will then be able to further question why they would recommend one course of treatment versus another.

Each of us will react differently to any one cure, and luckily there is rarely only one possible course of treatment. There is also a constant stream of new drugs and medical information which Health Professionals will be referring to. So the answer to 'What *can* be done?' will rarely be straightforward. This complexity may seem daunting, but we should remember that the Health Professionals are there to help us, and they should be able to guide us in finding the information we need to make the best decisions as we strive towards either recovering our health completely, or at least learning how to live with a certain medical condition or disability.

Louis K. had grown up in South Africa, and had spent most of his childhood playing out in the baking sun. He was white-skinned and in those days there had been little awareness of the need for sun-blocks to protect the skin. Later in his adult life he regularly went to a skin specialist who would check his skin for any pre-skin-cancer signs and if necessary the appropriate treatment was administered. This continued for about 30 years. Meanwhile he moved to live in Holland but regularly returned to South Africa. On one of his visits to his skin specialist in South Africa she noticed a lump under the skin on his left cheekbone, and was concerned that this might be an aggressive skin cancer. When Louis asked 'what can be done?', she advised immediate surgery, and since they might have to cut quite deeply this would be followed with some plastic surgery. Louis returned to Holland and took this analysis to his Dutch skin specialst. He asked 'what can be done?', and was advised that although surgery was possible it was not necessary for now as it did look dangerous. Since Louis had been going to his skin specialist in South Africa for 30 years he felt she would have a more accurate insight into his skin cancers. He therefore decided to go back to South Africa and have the operation. In this case she had been right, the cancer they removed was of a particularly aggressive type. Louis had asked "What can be done?" of two different Health Professionals, and was able to make an informed decision between them. He was also helped by using other questions on the PAC-CARD such as 'What should be done?'

TIPS – 'What can be done?'

* **Keep an open mind with this question, it is a tool to gather information.**
* **Since a course of treatment is often developed and decided upon over various appointments (as noted earlier) it is particularly useful to write down all suggestions and recommendations which arise from our meetings with Health Professionals.**
* **To have a clear list to later refer to, think about and discuss at one's ease is invaluable.**

5c. What should be done?

This question is attached to a time line and may or may not be urgent. It is important to find out at any point during our meeting with Health Professionals which actions need to be immediately taken or planned. For example, immediate medicine, blood tests, X-rays, MRIs, new appointments with other specialists, surgery...

It is a question which may also receive the answer, *"No immediate action is necessary."*

Sander R. had a physically demanding job, which over the years had caused recurring knee problems. During a visit to his knee specialist he mentioned that the arthritis in his hip was also becoming more and more painful. He asked: "What should be done?" and who he could go and see. His knee specialist, who by this time he knew quite well, reacted immediately by arranging for an X-ray of Sander's hip. When the results came back, he explained that the arthritis had developed considerably, and warned Sander that within a year at the latest he should have hip-replacement surgery. He told Sander to contact one of his colleagues to arrange the procedure. Over the next few weeks as Sander waited for his appointment to see the hip specialist, he became more and more stressed. He had already suspected that at some point it was likely he would have to have this operation. But he had thought that if at all, it would be in several years' time. He knew that a hip replacement was a major operation with a long recuperation period: how was he going to cope at home and worst of all what about his job? Would they, at such relatively short notice, be able to carry on without him... would he have to be replaced... once he was better would he get his old job back again... and would he even be able to do it once he had recovered from the surgery?

Three weeks later when he met with the hip-replacement surgeon he heard a completely different story. This specialist recommended that Sander wait a few years. The specialist said that he usually encouraged patients to make their own decision on when to have the operation, depending on how much pain or discomfort they were in and what they could live with. He explained that arthritis in the hip was a slow degenerative process and that it was usually best to wait as long as possible before operating, since this, in his opinion, would make no difference to the successful outcome of the operation. If Sander had been much older, there might have been more urgency, since an elderly patient would be less able to deal with such a major operation, but he was only in his mid-fifties. Sander later found out that his

*knee specialist 'liked to operate' and was well known
for recommending this as the preferred course of
treatment.*

*Sander decided that for him 'what should be done'
was... nothing dramatic. He just needed to live
with the pain until it was no longer tolerable. He
would repeat-appointment with the hip-replacement
specialist to monitor the arthritis, take painkillers
from time to time and meanwhile find out who else
in this field of surgery had a top reputation.*

TIPS – *'What should be done?'*

❋ When asking this question keep remembering
that we are looking for a practical answer.
An understanding of possible actions which really
NEED to happen.

❋ However frightening or upsetting a Health
Professional's advice may be, keep remembering
we always have a choice. They are giving us
advice and offering us help based on their
knowledge and experience. They are not
imposing a particular action on us.

❋ Even if we are in an emergency situation where
it is highly likely that the Health Professional's
expertise will be gratefully received by us, it is
worthwhile to still ask this question. In this way,
any possible *'automatic pilot'* actions by the

Health Professional can be interrupted with a few seconds of reflection.

* Depending on the size of the hospital, the time of day, or the department, Health Professionals may be very busy and have quite a time pressure on their shoulders. Finding clear answers to this question will help to keep decisions focused and help us keep on top of (often) confusing hospital processes.

5d. What is the (scientific) evidence for their suggestion?

As noted earlier, developments in innovative drugs, surgical procedures and other solutions for many medical problems are constant. The amount of new medical information which Health Professionals will need to keep on top of is formidable.

An ongoing question which we the patients will be confronted with is why one choice of treatment should take preference over another. Is it better to go for a solid, well-tried treatment or should we take the risk with a new approach? Any kind of development and progress requires some of us to agree to be the first ones. Whether it is using a new kind of man-made valve in our heart, a 'never-before' transplant, an extraordinary new kind of synthetic covering, a ground-breaking drug...the list is endless. And yesterday's discovery is tomorrow's standard procedure.

In most countries with medical developments there are stringent tests and medical trials which will usually happen before they are offered to the general public. What we need, when Health Professionals suggests a certain course of action, is a very brief understanding of why they have made that choice.

Health Professionals will have had a scientific education so this question is pragmatic and can be answered with facts and figures. However, most of us are not scientists. We will therefore want an answer which informs rather than overwhelms us. Asking straightforward questions will help us to get one.

*L*ena M. had recently gone through the process of finding out she had breast cancer and undergone a lumpectomy, followed by 5 weeks of radiation therapy. Although emotionally upsetting and physically tiring, the treatment went well. Both her two sisters and even her father had over the past few years discovered that they had breast cancer and had all undergone surgery. Surprisingly, Lena and her two sisters tested negative for BRCA1 and BRCA2. (BRCA1 and BRCA2 are human genes that belong to a class of genes known as tumour suppressors. Mutation of these genes has been linked to hereditary breast and ovarian cancer.) After the radiation therapy, Lena was advised to take the drug Tamoxifen on a daily basis, for at least two and a half years. Like most drugs, Tamoxifen has (sometimes unpleasant) side effects. Over the course of her cancer treatment Lena had had numerous discussions with different doctors, her sisters, other family members and certain friends who had also had cancer. She also read a lot of different information on the internet. Lena began to feel overwhelmed with so much information and remained undecided as to whether she should take Tamoxifen or not.

During the next meeting with her physician, although she had previously been given leaflets about the drug, she dared to ask the simple question, "What is the scientific evidence for your suggestion that I take Tamoxifen?"

The physician responded with a clear, to the point answer illustrated by a series of graphs, with enough focused information to help Lena decide to accept the advised treatment. Up to this moment Lena had been flooded with information together with experiencing the emotional rollercoaster of coming to terms with having cancer. When she asked this question in this *last meeting, it was in her own timing, she had space in her mind to be able to absorb and understand the evidence, and consequently she felt ready to make the decision to take the advice.*

TIPS – *'What is the (scientific) evidence for their suggestion?'* **The following kinds of questions will help to keep the answers simple:**

* **Is it tried and tested? If so for how long, and on how many people?**
* **Has the Health Professional used/done this before?**
* **If it is new, what medical trials indicate a switch to this method?**
* **If it has been used for a long time, are there any more recent medical solutions which could be more effective?**

5e. When will this happen?

It is so easy to either forget to ask this question or if the Health Professional gives us a time line, to not hear or remember the information. The question *'When will this happen?'* can refer to many parts of a process: when will the operation happen, the blood test, the appointment confirmation with another specialist...

Alice M., 18 years old, was taking a gap year and had decided to travel around part of Southeast Asia for 4 months. After 10 days in Thailand she came down with the inevitable tummy bug! She had a fever, diarrhoea and was vomiting for a few days and then it more or less passed, or so she thought. However, as she went on to travel through Laos and Cambodia she continued to feel weak and nauseous. After her amazing travels in the East she returned home to Amsterdam. Realizing that her symptoms were continuing and that she might have contracted some kind of infection she went to see her Doctor.

She arranged for Alice to have a blood test. The results came back negative. As her symptoms continued the Doctor told her to have a second round of tests, this time including testing her stools, but these test results were also negative. Alice's symptoms not only continued, but they seemed to increase. She was vomiting from time to time and feeling nauseous most of the time. After the second round of tests brought up negative results the Doctor sent her to the department of tropical diseases at the AMC (Academisch Medisch Centrum - a large Amsterdam hospital). Once again they did a round of tests and once again they could find nothing wrong with her.

Meanwhile Alice was becoming physically weaker and emotionally overwhelmed by living with such

unpleasant symptoms. She was also steadily losing
weight. The hospital agreed to run another round
of the same tests. After about a week Alice rang her
doctor for the results, but her doctor had heard nothing.

She waited and waited, trying to get on with her life.
Neither she nor her mother felt comfortable with
constantly ringing the Doctor. Since to date the
mystery of her illness had not been solved they had
begun to feel increasingly insecure about asking for
any more action from the medical profession. They
waited patiently. Weeks passed. It finally transpired
that in the last set of hospital tests they had indeed
found a rather common intestinal bacterium called
Helicobector pylori (a bacterium which is regularly
picked up by Westerners who travel in the East).
However, somehow the hospital had forgotten to
forward the results of the tests on to Alice's Doctor.
With all the delays that happened between each
test, waiting for results and re-testing as well as the
diagnosis being delayed by the last incident of the
hospital not forwarding the positive results on to her
or her doctor, it took more than 4 months for Alice to
receive treatment. Within about 10 days of a course of
very strong antibiotics, she finally began to feel better.
And after a few more weeks she returned to full health.
If Alice and her mother as a matter of course had
automatically kept asking the question: 'When will

the results of each test be known?' of all the Health
Professionals involved in this process, maybe that
final delay of many weeks would have been avoided.
It is very easy for us, the patients, to start to feel like
a bother to Health Professionals. Very often if there
is something wrong with our health, it will involve
medical tests and waiting for results. It is important
for us to understand the timing and be informed as
soon as there is information to be had, not only for
practical reasons but also for our emotional wellbeing,
since waiting for results can be upsetting if not out-
and-out frightening. Since we may not have been
through this particular process before, it is impossible
for us to know what is a 'normal' waiting time for a
set of results. If we can get clear 'timing' information
from Health Professionals *it is easier to also alert*
them if as in the case of Alice someone forgot to
forward the test results.

Sometimes Health Professionals can be precise with
their answer and sometimes this may not be possible.
"The operation will be scheduled to happen within the next
few weeks..." "...within six months' time..." "...will depend
on the availability of..."

It may also happen that the time frame(s) we are given
may change. It can be useful to specifically ask Health
Professionals how certain they are of their answer. If

many factors have to be in place before, for example, a specific operation can be performed, it could influence the certainty of the timing.

If you have received an unexpected diagnosis which requires immediate action, or for example you have been in an accident, then you will probably be in shock. This shock will be on several levels: if you have been physically injured, the shock will be physical as well as emotional. You may be further shocked on hearing that, for example, you immediately have to be operated on. Even in a non-accident situation, sometimes the pure fact of receiving concrete information about a proposed medical action can bring the shocking reality of our medical condition into sharp focus. At such times it is important to take mental space to accept or come to terms with this. It could be that in the meeting you ask for a couple of minutes to deal with your emotions. You may feel like crying, being angry or that you are just numb. But for that moment it will be hard to proceed with the conversation in any useful way. If you have a friend or family member with you, you might ask them to either comfort you or carry on the conversation for you.

It is also worth remembering that even if the Health Professional presents you with a certain timing for an operation or treatment it can always be changed, also by you. They may not like this and you may even be told that it is *'this date and time or never'*. But on further investigation it is amazing how often the so-called immovable appointment can be changed or the unavailable specialist can be contacted. It does however require that we the patients remain persistent, clear and positive.

It is also useful to remember that most hospitals are huge organizations with varying efficiencies in their organizational procedures. One department may be very professional and in the same hospital another could be quite chaotic, as in the case of Alice. And then with most medical procedures it will require several different departments coordinating their services. Once again, depending on the particular hospital, this can all too easily create delays in a promised timing.

As stated, when a Health Professional promises a certain time frame it is useful to ask how definite this is and if possible to enquire how many medical actions need to be in place for this to actually happen.

It could be that you are an inpatient in hospital and the nurse promises that you will see the surgeon that day. If you are anxious about the meeting and want to know what time to expect this, you could simply ask them to be more specific. If they cannot give you a more precise answer you could always ask them to let you know once they have a better overview of the timing. Hospital staff will probably be having to balance many people's needs and expectations so we need to remain sympathetic to the complexity of their responsibilities without going to the extremes of either accepting everything with a passive resignation or becoming overly demanding, frustrated or even angry. Neither are likely to benefit us. But we the patients need to make sure we are heard.

*B*etty R. (92 years old) was in hospital. She had severe abdominal pains and had been admitted for immediate tests including a colonoscopy (an internal examination of the large intestine). As the hospital was oversubscribed they had to put her in a side room off the maternity ward. The colonoscopy required that she did not eat anything after midnight of the previous day until after the test had been made. When she woke up, for the first couple of hours this was not a problem and Betty waited. She drank the water which she was allowed to drink and from time to time when a nurse passed by she enquired in a light and friendly way if they could find out when she would be given the internal examination. The nurses did not know, and since they were so busy rarely came into her room. Betty could see how overworked they were and did not want to cause a problem. She waited.

Midday came and went and the nursing-team shift changed. Betty slept a little and woke with stabbing abdominal pains. She rang for the nurse. Someone appeared who she had not yet met and who was not only surprised to see a 92-year-old in this room off the maternity ward but also knew nothing of her awaited medical examination. It finally transpired at 4.30 in the afternoon that the test had long ago been postponed until the next day due to an emergency treatment in the operating theatre. Since the message never got though to the medical staff looking after Betty, for no useful reason she did not eat for 22 hours. The consequence was that her health rapidly declined and she was too weak the next day to have the colonoscopy. She left the hospital a few days later, her health and strength having noticeably deteriorated due to this negligence. If Betty had dared to be more demanding and persistent in her questioning, this might not have happened.

TIPS – *'When will this happen?'*

✳ **If you receive information about the timing of a medical procedure which triggers an emotional response in you – this is normal. Give yourself time to recover your balance. This could mean asking for a glass of water and taking a few deep breaths to calm an adrenaline rush. Or asking for** your companion to take over your active role in the meeting.

* If for some reason the promised timing seems not to be happening, ask as soon as possible with clear warm determination if it has changed (as in the case of Betty).

* If you wish to have more time to re-consider the scheduling of a certain procedure TAKE IT. Find out what the consequences could be for postponing but resist feeling pressurized or bullied into action.

* If you have to wait, in your view, too long for an appointment, operation or other medical procedure, question further to understand why this is the case. Find out whether there is another way to solve this. For example by going to a different hospital or seeing another specialist.

5f. Who will do this?

This is another question that we all too often forget to ask. If we are talking to a surgeon about a certain operation it is easy to assume that they will be the one who will actually perform it. This is not necessarily the case. This can be upsetting if we have built a relationship of trust over several meetings and then hear that they will not perform the operation.

And sometimes at the last minute just before an operation the team changes due to, for example, an emergency elsewhere in the hospital. Or maybe the surgeon is sick – they are human too!

If we are a patient in an academic teaching hospital it may be that either part of our surgery, or even all of the operation is done by a student or junior doctor, under the supervision of the surgeon. Of course everyone has to learn, but depending on the complexity of our condition we the patients should be aware of who is doing what to our bodies and when appropriate be a party to the decision.

In some hospitals the patient will rarely be able to meet the surgeon who will perform the operation, for any length of time or even at all. Pre-surgery appointments are increasingly run by junior doctors or nurse practitioners. This is not necessarily a bad thing, as communicating information to patients is a big part of their job. A surgeon's skill is mainly focused on their particular area of surgical expertise, whether it is replacing heart valves or removing a cancerous portion of the liver. Being able to communicate with patients is often not part of their skill set.

Once you identify who the hospital proposes to perform a certain procedure or operation, find out as much as you can about them. If you have the opportunity, you could ask them directly about themselves. Otherwise try visiting the hospital website or even running a search of their name on the internet. Remember that if you are not happy with the choice you can ask for someone else.

Jane H. finally had the appointment with her surgeon. Although he seemed pleasant enough, as the meeting proceeded she began to feel less and less comfortable with the thought that this was the person who would operate on her. Throughout the meeting he was constantly picking at a small wound on his lip. He seemed altogether rather nervous, even in, for example, the way he picked up his pen to write a few notes. Since Jane had already had to wait a couple of months for her surgery, and did not want to upset anyone, she accepted the setup and the surgeon operated on her. Although the internal part of her operation seemed to go well, the way the surgeon sewed her up was clumsy and left her with a large unsightly scar. She later found out that he was on a temporary contract, which was not renewed. Jane learnt to live with the scar, but decided that if this ever happened to her again she would trust her gut feeling and ask for another surgeon.

Sometimes we may have already taken a dislike to someone due to the way they have talked with us during an earlier meeting. If possible, we need to form an opinion of their medical skills, independent of their skills as a communicator. They may even have pushed a button in us which had more to do with our past than to do with them.

On the other hand we may really like and *'click'* with a certain specialist and overlook the fact that they are not as qualified as we would like them to be when it comes to the operation.

Sometimes a hospital will book you to see the specialist in one appointment and their assistant in the next. Make sure that you understand why they do this so that you can decide whether to accept it or ask to see your initial specialist again. Very often the specialist will be part of a team. The team is more likely to work well if each person in the team is a skilled communicator, keep this in mind.

If you have asked enough questions and taken an active part in decisions, then, during the many vulnerable moments which are likely to happen, particularly right around the actual procedure, you will be able to feel more trust and therefore more relaxed with the medical team who are performing it.

It has been proven that the more emotionally and mentally at ease we are, the more chance our body has in responding positively to medical treatment. Rampant fear and anxiety are toxic.

TIPS – *'Who will do this?'*

* Be clear for yourself why it matters which Health Professional performs a certain task.

* Realize the range in the consequence with wanting to know which Health Professional is going to do what. Clearly there is a difference in importance between wanting to know *"Who is going to take my blood?"* and *"Who is going to operate on my heart?"*

* In a high-pressure, complex operation it could be useful to find out about the medical team who will perform the procedure. In the case of the promised surgeon becoming unavailable, who do they have in place as a back-up?

* If you are in a teaching hospital be clear about who you wish to operate on you. It is fine to state that you want a particular experienced expert, not a student.

* In some medical situations the members of the team can be as important to a successful outcome as any one specialist.

5g. Who is in charge of my welfare and treatment here?

Depending on what is wrong with us, once again this question could have several types of answers and may not need to be asked that often. All we the patients need to know, is who has the 'end responsibility' and who has the 'daily responsibility' for our treatment. It could be the same person. If we are seeing several different specialists it is always good to know which of them brings together and guides our process. In some countries the person who will have access to all our medical information will be our GP (general practitioner). By asking this question, we may also gain insight into how the hospital is structured in the area of roles and decision-making.

Jacqueline H's father, Wim, was admitted to hospital on a Saturday evening with a painfully swollen stomach. On the Sunday morning they ran some tests and X-rays and in the beginning of the afternoon the surgeon explained the results to the family (his wife and three daughters). Wim had a tumor blocking his bowels and should be operated on immediately. Using drawings and a whiteboard he explained that there were two options. They could place a stoma (a surgically created opening in the large intestine that allows the removal of feces out of the body, bypassing the rectum, to drain into a bag which is attached to the outside of the person's body). This his family immediately stated was not an option as Wim was suffering from advanced dementia and would most certainly keep trying to pull at and remove the bag which would be attached to the stoma. Or they could remove the tumour and hope that his bowels would then be able to regain their proper function. There was a chance that his bowel would leak. If this happened they could not operate again and Wim would not survive very long. When the family asked what would happen if they did nothing the surgeon said: "Wim must be operated on, otherwise he will die." Wim was therefore immediately prepared for surgery. As the family were waiting for him to be taken to the operating theatre the head of the intensive care unit came into the room and immediately asked the family lots of questions –

he was clearly very stressed. He informed them that since Wim also had a heart problem (everyone knew about this) he would most certainly be delirious after the operation and therefore impossible to nurse. He literally said, "What in God's name are you, as a family, doing?...there is a big question whether this man will even survive the operation and if he does he will end up in a nursing home... I do not want to have this man in my intensive care unit, after the operation we will wheel him back to

his room and then... we will see what happens!"
The whole family felt traumatized. Once they had
regained some emotional balance they talked
through all the options again; finally deciding on
no medical intervention they took Wim home. He
died peacefully a few days later. Once they started
to get over their anger and shock, Jacqueline and
her family realized that if they had asked the
question: '**Who is in charge of Wim's welfare and
treatment here?**' then maybe they would have
been able to discuss the different alternative actions
with a professional who had a wider perspective on
her father's wellbeing and impending death. They
might then, in a less traumatic way, have reached
the kindest decision: not to operate on a man in his
mid-eighties with advanced dementia, but to let him
peacefully die at home in the midst of his family.

TIPS – 'Who is in charge of my welfare and treatment
here?'
* **If we know who has end responsibility for
  our welfare in a certain medical institution or
  department it can be surprisingly empowering.**
* **Knowing if the person we are talking with has
  end responsibility will help us to know how much
  power they actually have to make a certain thing
  happen.**
* **In the event of dissatisfaction and the need to**

possibly instigate fast action it is essential to know who has the ultimate responsibility for our wellbeing.

5h. Who is my contact person, should I have any problems/further questions?

This may or may not be the same person as the individual who has end responsibility. It could be an assistant, and even someone we have never met. It may not be one particular person but just anyone from the particular department we are registered into.

If possible it is useful to have a precise name (and their job title) and to keep that name readily available. Be prepared to accept that the name which is given is not necessarily the person who will be able to answer a particular question. They may be the reference point, who will then be able to refer you to whoever is available at the time you ring or pass by.

Depending on the hospital and Health Professional we may be given a general reception telephone number or even an individual's mobile phone number. What is important for us is that we have an effective current telephone number readily at hand, should we ever *need* to ask for help.

TIPS – *'Who is my contact person, should I have any problems/further questions?'*

* Make sure when asking for a contact person that you also have a current telephone number for them.
* Know if a telephone number is the reception or if it will take you directly to the person who you wish to talk with.

5i. What must/can I do now?

Although Health Professionals are there to offer us their expertise, there are a surprising number of actions which we the patients can and must do ourselves. The first part of this question refers to immediate action and will probably be connected to procedural actions. It could be that we have to immediately have an X-ray and therefore have to take certain forms to another department and come back with the results, or have a blood test and ring for the results in three days, or make an appointment with another specialist through the receptionist as well as making a new appointment to see this specialist within two weeks...

We may also be told that we need to come back at some future date, such as in twelve months' time. Most hospitals would send a reminder for this, but it is useful to make a note anyway.

What can happen is that we become part of the administration procedures as we pass different forms back and forth. On the other hand in some hospitals they organize and coordinate all the actions and what we have to do is 'patiently' wait.

The other part of this question is to find out what we can do to keep our medical condition under control, or support a certain treatment. For example: after an operation it may be vital to walk every hour for a minimum of 10 minutes to avoid blood clots, or we should make sure when we take a prescribed medicine that we do not eat for one hour before taking it. We may need to make lifestyle changes, such as to stop eating salt or drinking alcohol, lie down every day for two hours minimum or repeat a certain exercise sequence. It could feel like a restriction or an imposition on our daily way of living. Or we could look at it as something practical that we can do to help ourselves. And in that way feel more empowered.

Jenny R. was in a car accident. She suffered whiplash and a broken arm which needed surgery. After the operation she asked what she could do to support her healing process. She was given the advice to regularly rest with her hand higher than her heart and once the wound started to heal, six times a day to put ice around the swelling for ten minutes. (Her arm was not in plaster, but was being held in place with the use of metal screws and a brace.) The nurse also gave her the tip to use (and re-use) a pack of frozen peas wrapped in a tea cloth, as this is a cheap and flexible way to apply ice to the body. Both these actions would increase her blood circulation around the operated area and consequently help the healing process. She then asked if there were any physical signs that she should look out for which might show if the wound was not healing properly. She was advised to check her temperature twice a day (at the same times) and make sure that it remained normal, regularly feel the temperature of her skin around the wound and note the colour of the skin. If it became hotter than the rest of her skin or changed colour and looked inflamed, and/or her temperature went up, this could mean that there was a slight infection. In which case she should contact her GP (General Practitioner). Jenny wrote these tips down and went home. As she was in shock it was not until a couple of days later, when she found the piece of paper she had written the advice on, that she remembered she could do something herself to help her recovery. It immediately made her feel a bit stronger emotionally and as the weeks progressed she saw that her actions with the ice and resting with her arm higher than her heart really made a difference

– the swelling decreased and it was less painful. By being able to pro-actively help her recovery Jenny felt more positive about coping with her injury. She also found that when she had her next hospital visit she was particularly perceptive about how her body was healing and could give the Health Professionals precise answers to their questions.

TIPS – *'What must/can I do now?'*

* Remember that in most cases there will be something that we either can or must do to benefit our health.

* The question what must/can I do may relate to helping in medical procedures by booking appointments etc, or to changing our behaviour.

* Make a note of any recommendations, advice or requests. It is easy to forget.

* If repeated daily actions are required, get your family or friends to help you remember.

* If you are required to take action in several months' time, immediately note it in your diary.

* If you have to take a combination of medicines at precise times of the day create an effective method to remind yourself – for example use a special pill box with sections for each day, use your alarm clock or mobile phone to bleep-remind you, ask a friend or family member to help you remember...

5j. If you do not understand something, ask for it to be explained, in another way, for example with pictures.

It is amazing how many of us do not dare to ask more questions when we do not precisely understand what a Health Professional is telling us about our health. For most Health Professionals what they describe to us will probably be something that they say many times within a week. For them it is often simple and obvious. Some Health Professionals will have been trained to explain complex medical facts to a wide range of people: from a patient who may be a biology teacher to another who may not know that they have a liver or what its function is. There are also many Health Professionals who will not have received training in this area of communication. In either case they will not have time to give us an anatomy lesson so it is useful to let them know as quickly as possible if there is anything we do not understand.

If we do not understand something there can be a tendency to feel stupid, vulnerable and helpless. If we feel even a shadow of insecurity it is useful to remind ourselves that it takes two to communicate effectively and the Health Professional may have been unclear, too complex or just talking too fast! Take a deep breath and...immediately ask them to explain in a different way, otherwise they may repeat exactly what they just said and we will be none the wiser. However, sometimes just asking what certain words mean and asking Health Professionals to speak a bit slower can make all the difference. For some of us complex medical terms and descriptions can make us feel confused about what is happening, in which case it can help to see a photograph or diagram to illustrate the explanation.

Pieter S. had been diagnosed with testicular cancer. His doctor had given him a detailed explanation of where exactly in his testicles the cancer was, what kind of cancer it was and the percentage likelihood of it having spread elsewhere in his body. The doctor gave a complex description of where a secondary cancer could occur and the kinds of operations, tests and drugs they would recommend. Pieter left the meeting understanding that a lot of awful things could be happening to him and that there would have to be a mass of medical procedures. In terror he walked out of the hospital imagining the cancer was multiplying itself around his body with each and every breath. Once home he realized that he had understood very little of what the doctor had said to him, the only thing that was ringing in his head was the dreaded word CANCER. After calming himself down he decided to ring a few friends, one of whom suggested that during his next appointment he could ask the doctor to re-explain his condition and this time use pictures or photographs. Pieter did just that. By asking the doctor to re-explain in a different way Pieter understood not only what was happening to him but what he could do to prepare himself for the decisions that would have to be made in the next months. He found out that a lot of what the doctor had described in the initial meeting were possibilities not facts about his specific cancer. By asking the doctor to describe the medical information in a way that he could understand, Pieter found that he was less frightened. It also helped him to be able to ask useful questions throughout his whole journey back to health.

Once we have the name and brief description of what may be wrong with us there may be a temptation to gather more information about it. As mentioned in section 4, the internet can be a fast and easy way to find out medical information. Remember that there is a lot of information on the internet which is inaccurate or untrue. We are not doctors and will probably not be able to see the difference. By all means use it as a way to understand more about your health but keep referring back to the Health Professionals as they will have access to your specific files and case. More information from other sources may help you understand what the Health Professional is telling you and may even give you the confidence to ask specific questions. It is sometimes supportive to use the internet to further understand how our body works as a whole and not necessarily connected to our own medical problem. Keep your questions simple and resist making a self-diagnosis!

TIPS – *'If you do not understand something, ask for it to be explained, in another way, for example with pictures.'*

* If you do not understand something that the Health Professional says to you it does not mean you are stupid. It just means you do not understand. It takes two to tango.
* It is to both yours as well as the Health Professional's advantage that you understand as much as possible about your condition. Therefore do not wait to say if you do not understand something. Time will be saved by you stating this immediately it happens.
* You may not understand something simply because you are in pain or are frightened and can therefore not listen well. Try to recognize if this is the case, or if the Health Professional is just being too complicated, technical or speedy!

5k. If surgery is recommended, ask how frequently they and/or the hospital perform this operation.

If surgery is recommended to us, our first reaction could range from relief to fear and panic. If we are in pain then the prospect of that ending could mean we gratefully accept any help offered. But we should still do all we can to ensure the help we receive is the best that is available. Surgery is a skill, which will generally improve with practice. This will hold true for an individual surgeon as well as a certain medical team and hospital facility. Depending on the complexity of the operation it is always best to know how often a surgeon and/or hospital performs the procedure.

Ideally, we would want someone who regularly performs this surgery. Practice makes perfect. If however your specialist does not have so much experience this may not be critical as long as the hospital and medical team involved have the desired experience. If neither exist it is worth finding out which hospitals near you do have the experience and expertise in the required area. If you are prepared to travel, you could also look further afield to see which are the best hospitals to go to for your particular condition. Very often different hospitals will have different specialties.

It is not an insult to ask Health Professionals these things. It is pragmatic and fact based. It is your body. But because of the god-like status of many specialists, it may be easier to ask a car mechanic who specializes in Citroëns if they can also fix the brakes on your car which is a Fiat! So it may help to think of it as a 'garage' question.

*S*imon P. had for a long time been suffering from acute tiredness so when he heard that his heart had a leaking valve which needed immediate surgery he felt a mixture of relief at knowing his tiredness was real (and not imagined as had been suggested by some people) and fear at the prospect of open heart surgery. The next day he found himself sitting in a consultation room meeting with a young female heart surgeon. He felt uncomfortable on two accounts. Firstly because she looked too young to have enough experience and secondly because she was a woman. He dared to challenge her expertise once he realized that she would be performing the operation. It turned out that not only was she older than she looked but she was top in her field, and he was lucky to have her as his surgeon! He later apologized for questioning her so aggressively; luckily she was used to such assumptions and had a sense of humour. She also said that she preferred a patient to ask these questions up front so that she could

either quell their doubts or recommend another
surgeon. She had no desire to operate on a patient
who did not trust her.

TIPS – *'If surgery is recommended, ask how frequently*
they and/or the hospital perform this operation.'

* To ask if someone has a lot of experience in
  something as pivotal as performing a certain
  operation on our body is a basic question. *It is*
  not personal.
* A surgical operation is a skill, which improves
  with practice. This is a proven fact.
* A medical operation is usually a one-off occasion.
  Once it is done it is done, it is not the same as
  asking for a second opinion.
* Time permitting, we should make sure that a
  surgeon, medical team and/or hospital have
  regular experience in performing the proposed
  operation.
* Do not assume (as in the case of Simon) that a
  doctor has or does not have certain hands-on
  experience. *Ask the question with open curiosity.*

5l. If you would like a second opinion, ask what the procedure is, who should you contact.

Very often a patient will not dare to ask for a second opinion as they do not want to anger or insult their specialist. The general feeling is that if we upset the specialist they will no longer have our wellbeing at heart. They may even turn against us! Most specialists will regularly be consulting and discussing medical cases with their colleagues and peers; two or more minds will often be better than one. If we have a particularly complex or tricky medical condition our specialist may have already discussed this with other professionals. If they have tried various medicines to no avail they may even themselves suggest that we visit another specialist or hospital for a second opinion.

So to ask to see someone else, particularly if we have doubts, insecurities or if little medical progress seems to be happening, is a logical step. It should not be seen as negative criticism. If we the patients do not mean it as criticism then we should try to make that clear by the tone of our voice and the way we word the question. If the specialist is defensive, it could be in response to the way we asked or they themselves may be feeling insecure. However, we are not responsible for their ego, and if it is a question of ego then they may not be the person we wish to continue to consult.

Most specialists are scientists and part of their desire and training is to identify and solve medical problems. Sometimes if they cannot make a clear diagnosis or cure certain symptoms they can feel disempowered. Once again that is their problem, we must try not to make it ours, and in the most graceful way possible find another specialist to help us. Sometimes by asking this question we can find out more about the curiosity and emotional maturity of our specialist and either gather more trained and talented minds together to tackle our medical problem or move our case on to meet with another hopefully more knowledgeable and/ or open-minded person.

A lex W. had an eye infection. His eyes were red, itchy and stinging. Each morning on waking his eyelids would be crusted together. When he first visited an ophthalmologist (eye specialist) she diagnosed conjunctivitis and gave him some eye drops, which she said should clear it up within the week.

This was not the case. Although the severity of the itchiness in his eyes reduced his eyes continued to be excessively watery with the slightest change in temperature or air current. The ophthalmologist tested for several eye conditions and found nothing. The only way she could reduce Alex's discomfort and symptoms was with some eye drops which contained cortisone.

Prolonged use of this could produce cataracts, eventually leading to blindness, so she checked his eyes every couple of weeks. After quite a few months and little change Alex proposed that he went to see another ophthalmologist. She readily agreed and suggested a colleague in one of the larger hospitals. At this hospital there were many more facilities and they quickly deduced that Alex had a type of blepharitis. Alex was advised to regularly clean the inside ridge of his eyelids with a certain medical tissue and from time to time put a warm flannel on his eyes. It was described to him as a chronic condition for which there was little else to be done. He regularly cleaned and looked after his eyes in the manner advised and found over time that most of his symptoms disappeared.

If Alex had not asked for a second opinion he might have continued taking the cortisone, the long term side-effects of which would have harmed his eyesight. On reflection he wished that he had asked for a second opinion a couple of months earlier.

TIPS – 'If you would like a second opinion, ask what the procedure is, who should you contact.'

✳ **It is reasonable to want to have a second or even third opinion to identify what is wrong with us as well as investigating what would be the best course of treatment.**

* Remember that in many medical setups Health Professionals will be working in a team, and will routinely discuss cases with each other. We can even ask: "Have you discussed my case with your colleagues?"
* Be sure to ask with the desire to find out more, rather than expressing a sub-text of dissatisfaction.
* By requesting a second opinion we will be able to see what kind of a scientist our specialist is. Depending on what we are suffering from it can anyway be useful to have more than one expert's analysis.

6. Write Main Facts Down

To write notes during a conversation with a Health Professional as well as continue the conversation can feel rude or awkward.

This may be because whilst we are writing there will have to be a pause in the talking. If you have a companion with you they can write notes for you, which can speed things up a bit. But it is worthwhile pausing to make sure they have written down the main points and it may also be useful for them to take part in the discussion. The Health Professional may also be writing notes from time to time, in which case we can make our own notes at the same time.

So what is the important information to write down and what can we leave out? If we are young and still at school or college, then taking notes during a class will be a daily activity. But for most of us this will not be the case. We need to develop our own way of briefly writing information, which we can actually understand once we read it later!

TIPS – *For writing notes*

It is useful to write down facts which might easily be forgotten. For example if any of the following topics are discussed:

* Specific names for an illness/condition.
* Names of medicines.
* Timing for any further treatment.
* Names of other Health Professionals we will have to meet.
* Names of other departments in the hospital we will have to visit.
* Names of other hospitals or medical facilities we may have to go to.
* Names of help organizations which we may wish to contact.
* The sequence of a certain procedure we may have to go through.

Your notes will have to be in shorthand. For example, if the specialist Dr Spasm is explaining that:

> '...the acute pain in your lower back has been diagnosed as a herniated disc. They can see from the MRI (Magnetic Resonance Imaging), which they took two days ago, that it is pressing on some major nerves in your back. These nerves lead to your legs, hence the pains in your leg. They believe that it is too bad to be able to only advise structured rest, exercise and physiotherapy. To avoid permanent

damage to the nerves leading to your legs and to stop the pain, they recommend surgery. This should happen as fast as possible and they wish to schedule it for within the next two weeks, they will be able to inform you within three days. Before the operation they will need to run a series of standard tests which are...'

Your notes may look like this:

Back Op. Urgent – Herniated disc – possible Nerve damage.
Advise - Op. within 2 weeks – get date in 3 days.
Pre-op:
Blood – today – 2nd floor phlebotomy dep.
MRI – next days – App. Arr. today through this dep.
Make App. With post op care. ask receptionist
Medicine same until op.
Surgeon Dr Spasm – expert – for him + team – routine op.

6a. Read them back to the doctor/health professional for them to confirm. "What you are saying is..."

Once everything has been discussed it is important to double-check the main points listed in your notes with the Health Professional. If you have incorrectly written down facts which you later refer to as correct it can cause unnecessary confusion and distress. Although it may take a minute or two longer it can save time later. If we start our double-checking with a phrase like *"What you are saying is...."* and then list the points from our notes, it means that we are showing the Health Professional what we have understood and giving them the opportunity to clarify or affirm. Either way we the patients will be more likely to feel we are actively taking part in the decision-making and medical process.

Janet P. had colon and liver cancer, and for the past 3 years she had regularly been in and out of hospital. During the course of her treatment she learnt, at the end of each meeting, to repeat back in her own words what the Health Professional told her should happen next. Whilst doing this she could also add any observations she had to their preferred course of action. After one course of treatment her radiologist advised that the next course of action was: "to wait and see what happens." By repeating his proposed next course of action back to him using the 'what you are saying....' format, Janet was also able to remind him of what happened last time: "...last time you also advised 'to wait and see' and the tumor grew very rapidly". The radiologist then remembered the earlier occasion and changed his advice. Janet realized that since the doctors saw so many

patients they did not always remember the details of her individual case. No doubt some are more conscientious than others, or better at remembering, but they almost certainly will not have time to read our entire file from beginning to end before each appointment. Janet felt that this way of summarizing and questioning would
"...jog their memory, making me less of a number and more of an individual case and person".

We do not need to leave this kind of cross-checking until the end of the appointment. If we feel the information is confusing or complex we can use the structure: *"What you are saying is..."* from time to time throughout the appointment.

I have found that when I use this approach during an appointment, Health Professionals start to be more exact and clear in the way they talk to me.

TIPS – *Read your notes back to the doctor/health professional for them to confirm. "What you are saying is..."*

✳ **By using the phrase 'What you are saying is...' we can not only check our own understanding but we can give the Health Professional a moment to reflect on their own advice, or maybe correct any misunderstanding.**

* If we use this form of questioning from time to time throughout an appointment it can make it easier to stay on top of understanding complex or unfamiliar information.
* It is a quick way to check the accuracy of our notes.

6b. Remember to keep your notes carefully and if necessary, over time, refer or add to them.

This seems so obvious but it is all too easy to forget to take paper and pens with us and to have them at hand at all times if we are staying in hospital. Or if we do remember to take them, we may find that with all the other new and sometimes worrying things we have to negotiate and remember, we leave the notes somewhere, never to be found again. These pieces of paper with all our important notes from a medical appointment simply get mislaid. We may even, half-consciously, deliberately lose them, since we are probably wishing this was not happening to us...

This is why it is useful to either buy a small notebook or have an envelope or file that we always put our notes in. Sometimes there may be a gap of several months between one appointment and another. Sometimes we believe that we will not have to return to see the specialist ever again and months later something un-expectedly happens and we have to go back to see them. There can be many reasons to keep all our notes together in one place, sometimes for years.

On the top of the page of any appointment notes, or any other time when you have met with a Health Professional (for example if you are an in-patient in hospital), **remember always to date it and name the person you talked with**.

These notes can also be invaluable when we are talking with several different Health Professionals. In this way we can immediately refer to the exact person who advised a certain course of action and accurately describe what they recommended and when. It could be something as simple as the hospital catering giving you certain food which when you double-check with your notes you can clearly confirm should be something different, such as a salt free diet.

Another reason why it is useful to keep these brief notes in the form of a log book (with dates and names) is that all too quickly the simplest of complaints can become more complex. Since with most western medicine, hospitals are divided into departments which focus on different parts of the body, as mentioned previously, we may have to visit several different departments or even hospitals. Although the hospital may understand its own structure (we hope), for us it can become confusing. Sometimes writing a brief and clear log book helps us to understand this complexity. Maybe by re-reading it we can revisit, understand and even re-evaluate decisions.

It also means that when we discuss what is happening to us with friends and family we can be precise, and everyone gets similar information. And should we receive advice from people other than Health Professionals then at least it will be based on sound information. It is surprising how easily people who are not professionals offer advice which is reacting to the patient's inaccurate information. This can get out of hand and sometimes even be harmful. Fear in such situations can multiply dramatically from the smallest misunderstanding or exchange of misinformation.

John B. had been supporting his wife through three major operations, over a period of approximately two years. Several months after the first operation it became clear that it had not been totally successful. And under the recommendation of a new surgeon a second operation was planned. This too, for various reasons, not only failed to solve his wife's back problem but led to an infection in her backbone around the site of the surgery. A third operation was then performed to try and remove the infection caused by the second surgery. His wife, who throughout the whole time was in continuous pain, had lost 16 kilos and was steadily getting weaker and weaker. The pressure on both of them was immense. What had started as a rather standard, although complex operation was turning into a nightmare. One of the ways that John navigated this escalating situation was to take notes during discussions with the surgeons and their teams. This not only helped him keep a handle on the situation but it also gave him a solid structure to refer to. He recounts that at one point the hospital was taking blood tests every day and then meeting with them to discuss the results. During one of these meetings he noticed the doctors were giving him and his wife contradictory information. By referring back to his notes he could see that this was indeed the case. So with the added confidence that his notes gave him, he brought this fact to the attention of the surgeons. At first they did not like the suggestion that they might be making a mistake, but as John could pragmatically refer to his notes they eventually took his observation seriously. They all looked again at the blood test results and came to a different conclusion, which led to a different course of treatment.

John noticed that after this incident the Health Professionals took him and his wife's comments more seriously.

The more practical and accurate we the patients can be when discussing our medical problems by referring to our notes the easier it is for others to help and support us – our friends and family as well as the Health professionals.

TIPS – *'Remember to keep your notes carefully and if necessary, over time, refer or add to them.'*

* **Even with the seemingly smallest complaint, become comfortable with writing down core facts during a discussion with Health Professionals.**
* **Either use a log book as described at the end of this publication or make sure you keep all your notes in a place which you can easily remember and have access to.**
* **Make sure that any meeting notes are dated and the health Professionals are named.**

....

....

....

....

....

....

....

....

....

....

....

....

....

....

7. Do Not Leave Or End the Meeting Until You Are Clear About What Happens Next

As long as we understand what happens next, then when we leave a meeting we will be less likely to loose our way within the medical process or institution.

It is important to realize that we will probably not fully understand everything that is discussed during our conversations with a Health Professional. Many times we will be building on an understanding as well as a realization of what we may have to cope with in the future, in connection to our health. These interactions can be packed full with information, decisions to be made and strong emotions so it is all too easy as we leave to suddenly think *'What next?'* It can be surprisingly easy to not really hear or listen to the last instructions of the Health Professional as we leave the room and the door closes behind us.

During a hockey tournament 16-year-old Ben skidded and fell, there was a resounding crack and pain shot through the left side of his body. Luckily his father was there watching the game and immediately drove him to the emergency department of the nearest hospital. It was not too busy and they only had to wait about an hour. After briefly examining his arm and shoulder the doctor asked his assistant to organize for Ben to have this area of his body X-rayed. Ben and his father found the X-ray department, which was located on another floor and wing of the hospital, and waited in line. After about half an hour Ben had the X-ray. They left with a feeling of relief and walked straight off down the corridor, returning to the original waiting room to see the doctor for the results. They waited another 95 minutes and when it finally came to their turn, found out that they were waiting in the wrong place. After the X-ray they should have gone to the plaster cast department where they were supposed to meet another doctor. It was there that the X-ray would be explained and the type of plaster cast would be discussed, decided on and immediately applied. They were not sure if the nursing staff had told them where to go after they left the X-ray department, but they were both exhausted, in shock and had not been asking after each part of the process: "What happens next…?"

This resulted in a long and distressing process becoming even longer and more distressing as pain and anxiety got mixed up with anger and frustration.

TIPS – *'Do not leave or end the meeting until you are clear about what happens next.'*

* After all conversations, meetings or interactions with Health Professionals get into the habit of asking *"What happens next?"*
* The 'time-line' answers to this question can be both long term and short term.
* If the answer is a longer time-line write it down *(e.g. app. in 3 weeks).*

The Author

Jessie Gordon was born and grew up in London. After studying Theatre and Performance at Dartington College of Arts, in south-west England, she worked for almost ten years as an actress in avant-garde theatre, most notably with the Pip Simmons Theatre Group, performing throughout Europe. She moved briefly into the world of music, playing the bass guitar in the rock band Flex, before going to live in Amsterdam, the Netherlands, where she has been resident ever since. Overlapping with her work in the performing arts Jessie developed a career as an illustrator/cartoonist for newspapers, magazines, postcard series and books, and also as a visual artist exhibiting in London, Tokyo and various locations in the Netherlands. More than twenty years ago, motivated by her ongoing exploration of the art of communication, Jessie co-created the company Executive Performance Training (EPT) www.executiveperformancetraining.com of which she is managing director to this day. Based in Amsterdam, EPT specialises in compact personal development programmes which connect the knowledge and techniques of effective live communication with: leadership, diversity and cross–cultural collaboration. These programmes take place in Europe, North America, Asia and Russia.

In 2013 Jessie's Book *What Gap? – A Communication Tool Box* was published. (Levboeken Publishers)

In 2011, prompted by her own hospital experiences with both a broken ankle and a lung embolism, Jessie developed the PAC-CARD (Patient's Action Communication card) and sponsored the creation of www.pac-card.com, which offers a 'free-download card' containing a checklist of essential support questions, for patients to use in any interaction with Health Professionals. To date this is available in 8 languages.

In 2012 Jessie wrote the book *The Patient's Guide - Think Ask Know* which explains how to effectively use the PAC-CARD. This was published in Dutch *Zo praat je met je arts* (Kosmos Publishers) in 2013.

Jessie has two children and lives in Amsterdam, the Netherlands with her Dutch partner.

My Log Book – *example*

Hospital/Clinic: ....

date: .... time: ....

....

Name of health professional: ....

....

Remember to Include Names of: *illnesses, medicines,*

procedures, appointments, hospital departments, people:

....

....

....

....

....

....

You have a medical appointment or
You are admitted to hospital.

Perhaps you are feeling anxious, intimidated, insecure, or even angry.
Perhaps you are confused as to what is going to happen and how
things work. This is completely normal.

Of course it is better to stay calm so that you can:

> **THINK** clearly
> **ASK** questions
> **KNOW** people are listening to **YOU**

The questions on this card can help you with this.
Use them in any meeting you have with a doctor/health professional.

**Explain to the doctor/health professional that you are using this card
as a checklist to help you communicate in a more effective way.**

**If you understand what is happening and why, you are also in a
position to actively help your own health related quality of life.**

1. **Take someone with you**
   - Whenever possible **it is useful to have someone with you,
     who knows you** and can also remain objective.
   - **Introduce your companion**, and say that they will be helping
     you understand, remember the meeting and also ask
     questions if they need to.

2. **Give information to any doctor/health professional
   you have not met before**
   Do not assume they already know:
   - **Your age, profession and social background**
   - **Your recent/relevant medical history** including allergies
     and medication.

3. Ask Questions to a doctor/health professional you have not met before (& Google them)

- How long have you worked here and what is your role/function?
- Do you have access to all my medical records?
- If I want to see them, how do I get access to my medical records?

4. Describe only your symptoms

- Make notes before hand to refer to.

5. Discuss all of the following points during the meeting:

- What is the problem?
- What can be done?
- What should be done?
- What is the (scientific) evidence for their suggestion?
- When will this happen?
- Who will do this?
- Who is in charge of my welfare and treatment here?
- Who is my contact person if I have any problems/further questions?
- What must/can I do now?
- If you do not understand something ask for it to be explained in another way, for example with pictures.
- If surgery is recommended, ask how frequently they and/or the hospital perform this operation.
- If you would like a second opinion ask what the procedure is, who should you contact.

6. Write the main facts down

- Read them back to the doctor/health professional for them to confirm "What you are saying is..."
- Remember to keep your notes carefully and if necessary, over time, refer or add to them.

7. Do not leave or end the meeting until you are clear about what happens next

WWW.PAC-CARD.COM ©Jessie Gordon, Amsterdam 2014,

This is a non-commercial initiative by EPT | www.executiveperformancetraining.com

Colophon

© Jessie Gordon, Amsterdam 2014

Design: Mulder van Meurs, Amsterdam

ISBN 978-1-326-06438-9

For reasons of privacy certain names in this book have been
changed.

Made in the USA
San Bernardino, CA
05 July 2015